ONCE UPON A REMEDY

Other books by Viviane Kolp

The Love of Life (poetry)

Medicine That Kills

Once Upon A Remedy

Canadian Cataloguing in Publication Data

Kolp, Viviane, 1957 -
    Once Upon A Remedy

ISBN 0-9680085-3-4

    1. Traditional Medicine. 2. Naturopathy. 3. Self Medication
I. Scheuer, Yvette, 1932 -   II. Title.

RC81.K64 1999   615.8'82   C98-901296-4

Cover Design by: Guy Ledoux
Cartoon Illustrations by: Diana V. Van Baaren
Typesetting by: Le Print Express, Vancouver, BC, Canada
Printed and bound in Canada by: Transcontinental Printing
Distributed by: Hushion House Publishing Limited

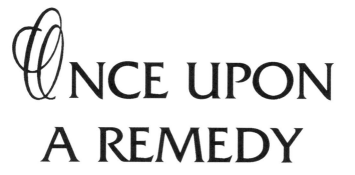

ONCE UPON A REMEDY

by
Viviane Kolp
and
Yvette Scheuer

Cartoons by
Diana V. Van Baaren

Cover Page by
Guy Ledoux

This book is dedicated
to all those who have
confidence in the healing
powers of nature's wonders.

Remedies that cure
must be toxin free
and pure

Important, please read:

The information in this book is intended to increase your awareness of preventive health care. By no means is it intended to diagnose or treat your medical problem or ailment. The regimens throughout this book are recommendations, not prescriptions, and are not intended as medical advice. Any decision you make involving the treatment of your illness is your responsibility and should include the guidance of either a doctor of your choice or a professional health counsellor, especially if you have a specific physical problem or are taking any medication.

Table of Contents

Introduction

It is essential to be self-sufficient in food and health. Too often nature is taken for granted. Too often we forget how abundantly it provides us with riches beyond all measure.

As human beings, we have the ability to be self-sufficient so it is essential to return to our original state of nature. Neglecting to do so will affect our emotions and intellect and will ultimately result in ill health.

Good health just doesn't take care of itself and is most often neglected by assuming that it will. By the time most people become aware that good health is the essence of life, they've already lost it.

The Earth was given to the human race and we who occupy it are bound to its surroundings. The all too common sun, water, air and sky to us make up an open paradise. If we exist in conjunction with nature, why not heal naturally? Just as we come into the world naturally, we die naturally. We all have the moral decision, without outside influence, to choose one method in preference to another. While generations of people come and go, Earth is forever here to stay. Let us be grateful to and respect Nature for it protects us in more ways than one.

I do not disclaim scientific knowledge or its technology, but I find that people have become so influenced by its alleged authority that they rarely question its shortcomings. It is human nature to self-destruct so we need to question man's lack of compassion to man???

Science claims to have improved so much so why is it that to this day it has failed to find a cure for the common cold? Why is it that people don't feel any better than they did twenty or thirty years ago? Science is strong, but it cannot defeat the powers of Nature!

"Science ought to be regarded as a tool."

"Nature does not betray thee whose heart loves and respects it".

In the process of studying and researching natural remedies, I became captivated by their effectiveness. The remedies in this book have been gathered by countless indigenous people from cultures around our planet and I thank all of them for sharing them with all of us.

Chapter I

Beauty Hints

Age Spots
Brittly Fingernails
Complexion
Dandruff
Eyelash Thickener
Hair Cleanser

Puffiness (of the face)
Skin Irritation
Stained Smoker's Finger(s)
Teeth Whitener
Warts

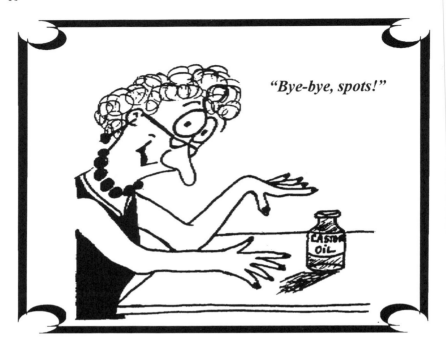

"Bye-bye, spots!"

LOOKING A WEE BIT SPOTTY, ARE YOU?

Perhaps age is catching up with you and so are those nasty brown spots; also called liver spots.

Rubbing castor oil well into the skin, morning and night, will take care of it. Within a month the spots should clear up.

The same method has proven to be successful with moles.

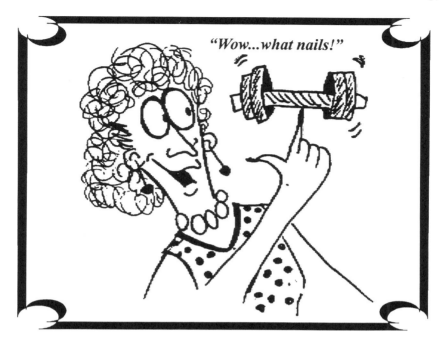

FRAGILE AS AN EGGSHELL

For brittle fingernails:
Before bedtime, massage your fingernails with a mixture of warm olive oil
and lemon juice. Rub in thoroughly and
wear cotton gloves overnight.

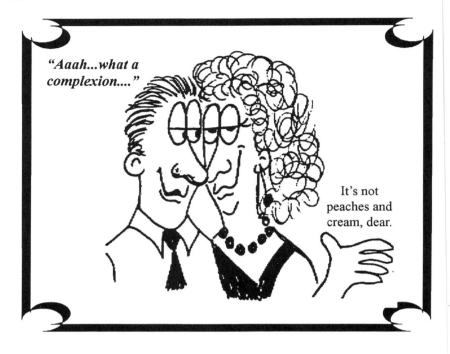

WHAT A COMPLEXION!

If you want to hold on to that healthy glow; cook an apple in milk, crush and apply when warm for about 20 minutes. When done, rinse away with cool water.

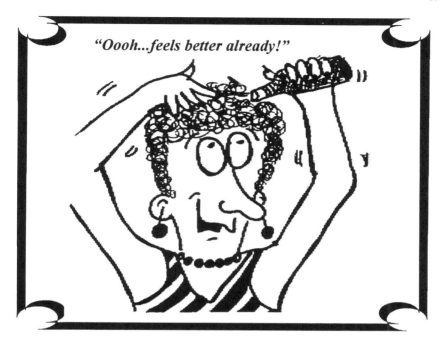

"*Oooh...feels better already!*"

I SURE WISH I KNEW HOW TO GET RID OF THIS FLAKY, WHITE STORM OF MINE!

Here's to your rescue!
Lightly warm up a cup of apple cider vinegar. Slowly pour onto your head and massage well into your scalp. Go about your business and wash out after an hour or so. Repeat a couple of times a week or until problem has cleared up.

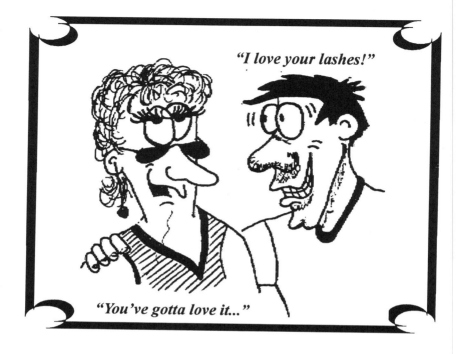

WHAT EVER HAPPENED TO YOUR EYELASHES?

To help thicken your lashes, gently rub either castor, linseed or Vitamin E oil on your eyelashes and into your eyebrows before retiring for your beauty sleep.

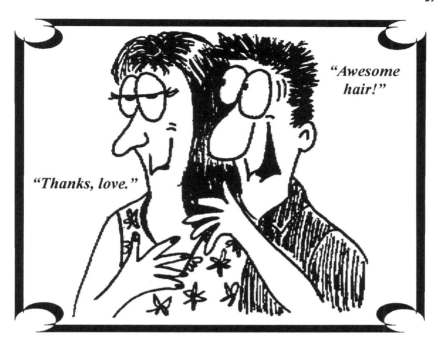

TIRED OF YOUR LIFELESS HAIR & HIGH-PRICED CONDITIONING TREATMENT?

Here's a penny's worth of secret your hairdresser won't share with you.
Next time you shampoo your hair, add a half teaspoon of baking soda. When done, rinse out and use your usual hair conditioner, rinse again and voilà! Clean, shiny, lusty hair!

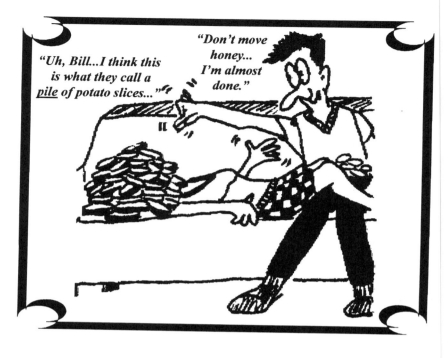

HANGOVER OR NOT...
SOME PEOPLE CONSTANTLY WAKE UP
WITH A PUFFY FACE

Trust me, this is no laughing matter. No one likes to be stared at for the wrong reasons.

Well, here's some help, assuming you don't mind getting up with the early birds.

On your face, apply a good layer of thinly cut raw potato slices.

Relax for a bit, then rinse off and voilà!

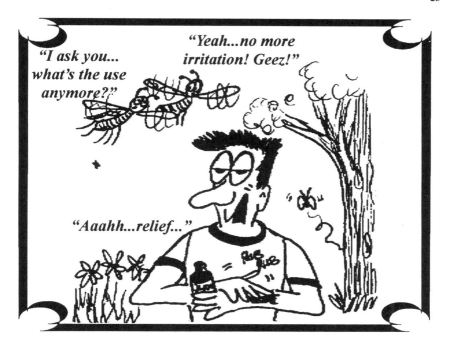

STOP RUBBING YOUR ARM LIKE THIS. YOU'LL ONLY MAKE IT WORSE.

Easier said than done!
For redness of the skin caused by minor irritation, apply any of the following to the irritated area: fresh cucumber juice; olive oil; or sweet almond oil. Gee, thanks for the choices!

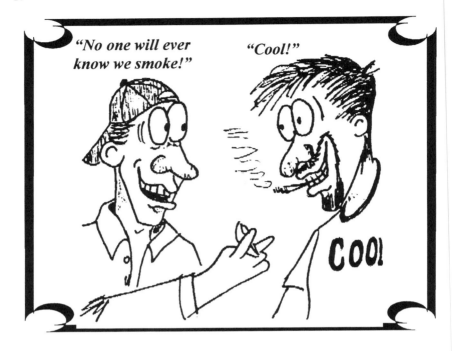

CAUGHT SMOKING!

For finger(s) stained by nicotine from smoking, rub your finger(s) regularly with fresh lemon wedges.

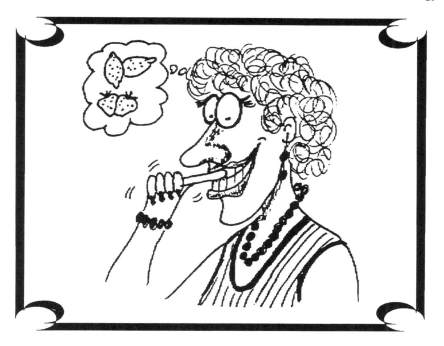

WHAT A SMILE!

To clean and whiten teeth, brush your teeth with fresh lemon juice, or its zest, once a week. If you can't stand the bitter taste of lemon try a mashed strawberry and brush away those stains (tastes berry good).

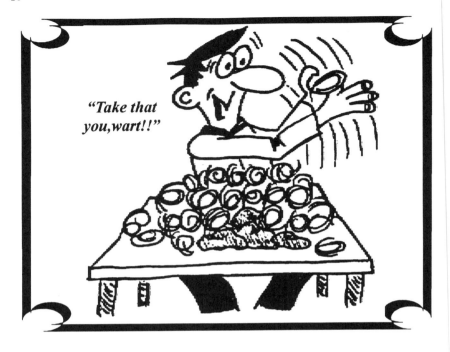

"Take that you,wart!!"

WAR ON WARTS

There must be as many homespun cures for warts as entries in the medical dictionary. But for a few wise men only one thing banished them...potato peelings. Rub the inside of the peel on the wart(s) several times a day and watch the lumps disappear. Warts are persistent because they are caused by a virus and potato skins are thought to contain antiviral compounds.

Chapter II

Skin Outbreaks

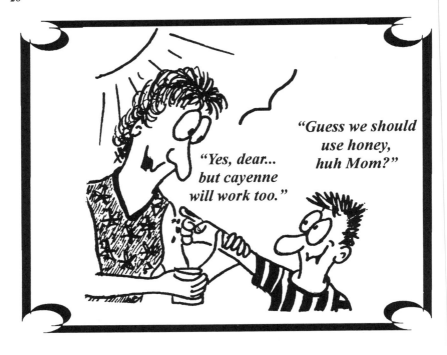

WHAT A BLOODY MESS! DON'T PANIC...IT'S ONLY A SMALL CUT.

For those nasty little nicks that bleed on and on...believe it or not, sprinkling a bit of cayenne pepper on it will stop the bleeding and without any burning sensation.

Honey works just as well and it contains antiseptic properties.

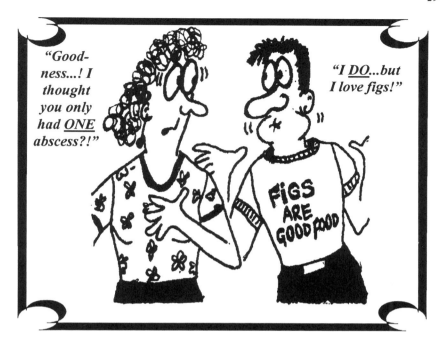

TELL ME IF I'M WRONG...BY THE LOOKS OF IT, YOU'RE CHEWING A LITTLE MORE THAN YOU CAN SWALLOW!

Wrong. This is no laughing matter.
I have a gum abscess*. Any ideas, smarty-head?
Try this: in lukewarm water, cook half of a fresh fig. When slightly cooled off, apply directly to the abscess.
Thanks buddy. What a relief!

*Abscess: swelling containing pus. Healing usually occurs after it drains or is opened.

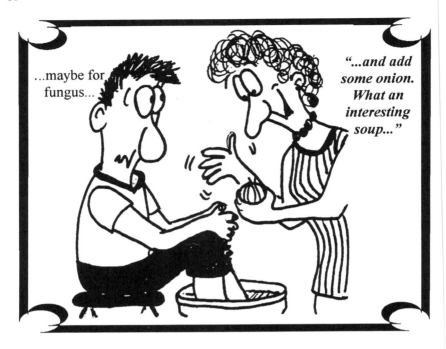

MAN! HOW OFTEN HAVE I TOLD YOU NOT TO WALK BAREFOOT IN PUBLIC BATHING OR SHOWER AREAS?! I SURE FEEL SORRY FOR YOUR FEET!

Here's something for your recurring Athlete's foot problem. Either choose to rub some onion juice between your toes several times daily or bathe your feet and add apple cider vinegar to the water. Repeat as often as necessary. Both these recipes will help clear the condition and discourage fungus from making a comeback. Eh!..one more thing....be sure to wear clean socks every day.

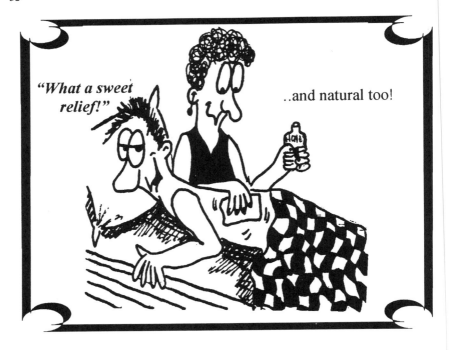

FOR HEAVEN'S SAKE...LET ME HELP YOU TAKE CARE OF THOSE AWFUL BEDSORES!

First, one must keep the affected area clean. Therefore be sure to arrange a daily sponge bath using Vitamin E soap.

Now, to start the healing process, apply some raw honey and cover with a clean dressing. Also, make sure the person wears loose-fitting cotton clothing and have someone help them move around in order to stimulate circulation. Another helpful idea to speed up the healing process is to drink a glass of water with a tablespoon of organic apple cider vinegar and a teaspoon of honey mixed in. Sip this with lunch and dinner. It will restore your pH level. In other words, the measure of acidity or alkalinity in your body.

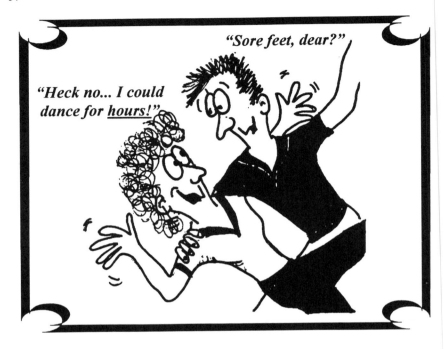

"BLISTERS" WHAT A PAINFUL PRICE FOR WEARING NEW SHOES

First sterilize a needle with rubbing alcohol, then make a small hole to release the fluid from the blister. When done, apply some honey and cover with a sterile dressing and watch it heal in no time. Honey is a natural antiseptic.

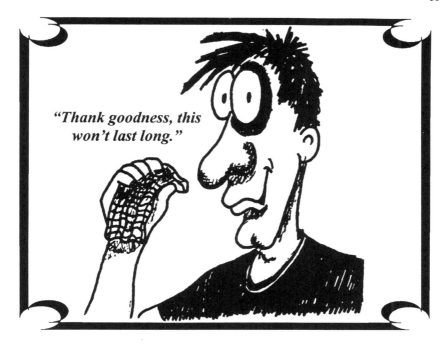

"Thank goodness, this won't last long."

I'M SORRY TO SAY THIS, BUT DID SOMEONE USE YOU AS A PUNCHING BAG?

To speed up the healing of those rainbow coloured bruises, simply use a clean cloth drenched in witch hazel solution and apply as often as required.

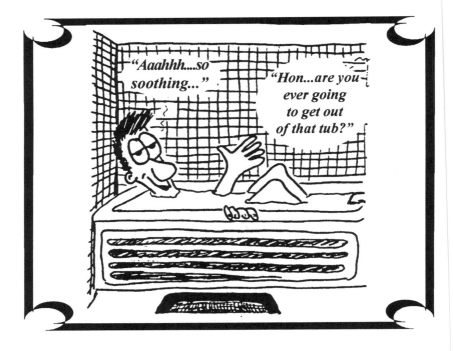

LOOKS LIKE A NASTY BREAKOUT!

Perhaps a food allergy or even a drug allergy? Maybe the heat, the cold or even sunlight? I don't know, just please get me something to rid myself of this itchiness. To relieve your discomfort, how about soaking yourself in a cool water bath with a little baking soda added to it. If this is not possible, get a dish and mix some baking soda with a little water until you've got a paste then apply it to the troubled area. "Relax, will you? The itching will subside."

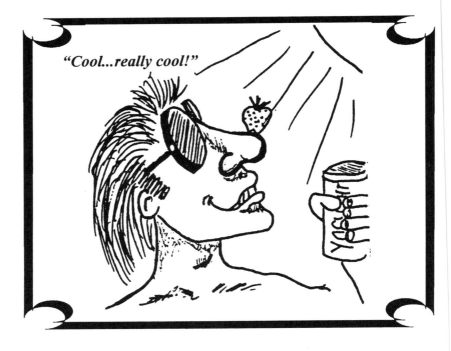

FEELING THE HEAT

Each summer, sunburns claim many victims. Here is an effective remedy after an overdose of ultraviolet rays. Mash a bowl of very ripe strawberries with equal quantity of plain yogurt then spread it evenly over the affected area, leaving it on for at least 15 minutes.

The active agent may be tannin in the strawberries. Tannic acid, a mixture of tannins, is used in the treatment of burns.

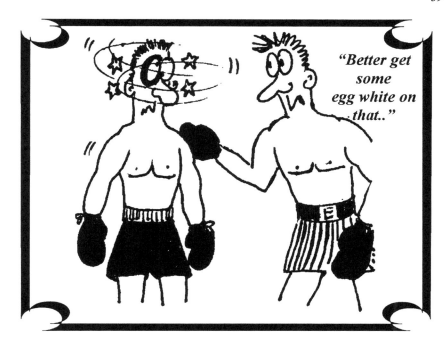

SURE LOOKS LIKE YOU'VE TAKEN ONE TOO MANY HITS! EITHER THAT OR YOU'RE A WEE BIT CLUMSY.

To bring down swelling caused by bruises, whip one egg white until firm and then gently massage onto the swollen area.

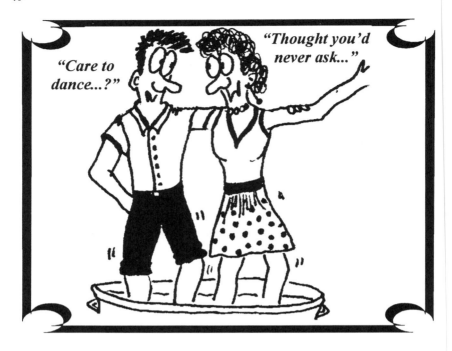

IF YOUR FEET KEEP ON SWELLING LIKE THIS, YOU WON'T BE GOING DANCING ANYTIME SOON.

Here is something worth trying and if the shoes fit...you'll be on your merry way...

For swollen feet, simply prepare yourself a foot bath to which you'll add some salt and vinegar.

Quit complaining, will you and just do it!

Chapter

III

Winter Blues

Bronchitis

Chapped Lips

Cold Feet (first remedy)

Cold Feet (second remedy)

Coughing Spell

Influenza

Sinus Inflammation

Sluggishness

Sore Throat

Tonsillitis

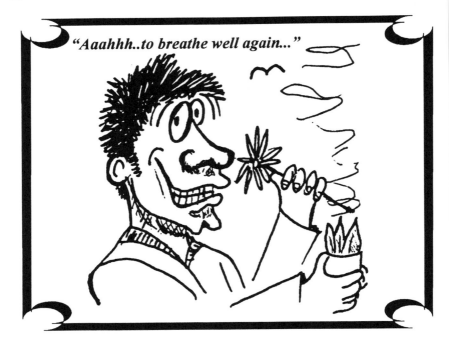

"*Aaahhh..to breathe well again...*"

CAN'T BREATHE?
NEED SOME FRESH AIR!

Smokers are not the only ones to experience coughing and breathing difficulties or bronchitis.

The condition is also aggravated by air pollution and cold weather. But a mild onset of bronchitis can be alleviated with laurel. It's been recommended to put two or three leaves of the herb in a

cup of boiling water for ten minutes
then add a teaspoon of honey and sip
slowly.

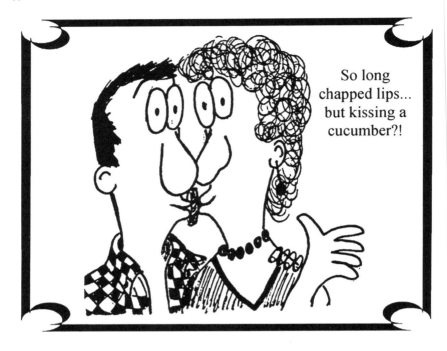

So long chapped lips... but kissing a cucumber?!

SORRY, BUT NO KISSY-KISSY FOR YOU TODAY!

For chapped lips, gently rub your lips with fresh cucumber slices several times a day until the problem is eliminated.

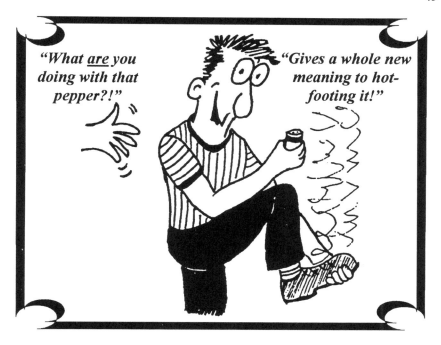

GEE WHIZ, I DON'T THINK I CAN BEAR MY COLD FEET ANY LONGER!

Well my friend, worry no more! Simply rub your feet with a little cayenne pepper powder, then on go your socks and boots (or shoes). Now that you're ready and warm, enjoy your day. Please be sure to avoid any eye or facial contact with the cayenne powder. It could prove to be irritating. So, play it safe and wash your hands after the pepper application.

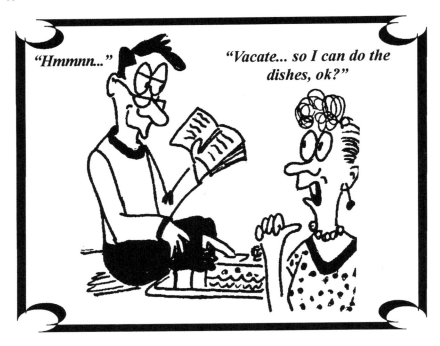

WARM HEART -- COLD FEET
SHIVER NO MORE

Here's for a speedy recovery.
Sit down and enjoy your favourite TV.
program, read a book or listen to music
while you bathe your feet in a basin of
warm soapy, bubbly water.
A little trick that will warm you up from
head to toe...or in this case toe to head.

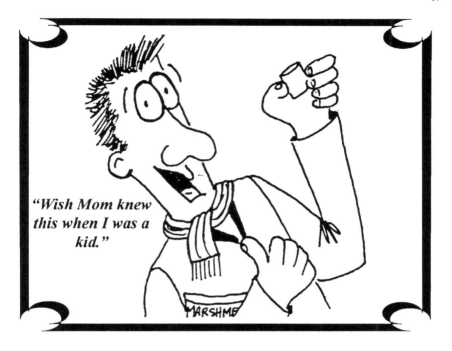

"Wish Mom knew this when I was a kid."

CAN'T STOP COUGHING?!

Get a hold of some marshmallows. Yes! The mucilage (viscous substance or sticky material) of those creamy, white puffs can actually soothe throat irritation and help you stop coughing.

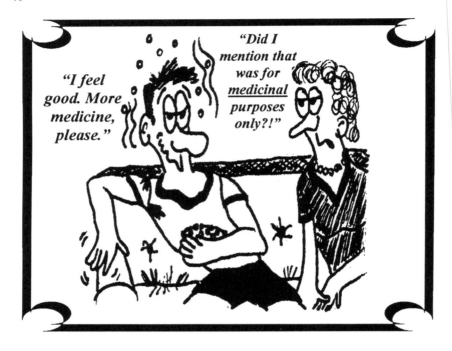

FALLEN VICTIM OF THE FLU (INFLUENZA)? HAVE I GOT A DESSERT FOR YOU!

Cherry Wine: Cover one kilo of either fresh or dried pitted cherries in red wine and add plenty of sugar (about one cup). Then cook for approximately twenty minutes or so. When done, serve this delectable dessert to your flu-stricken friend. Mm, mm, good...suddenly you feel much better.
*Do not consume if you have a fever.

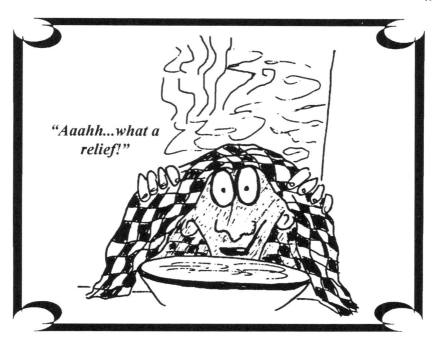

"Aaahh...what a relief!"

HAVING DIFFICULTY BREATHING? COULD BE THAT DARN SINUS INFLAMMATION AGAIN!

To ease discomfort: boil half a kettle of water then pour in a bowl and add a few drops of eucalyptus oil. Place a towel over your head and inhale for a few minutes. When done, splash your face with cool water to close facial pores. Repeat this action two or three times during the day.

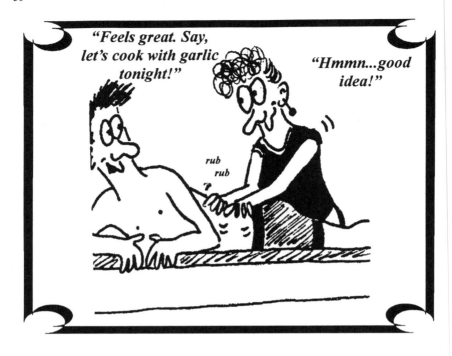

TIRED - WEAK?

Missing another day at work?
This has got to stop. Here is something
that will get you up and moving. Mix
two parts olive oil with one part finely
grated garlic then have someone use
this blend and give you a lower back
massage. Nothing like a little pamper-
ing to wake up those sleepy senses.

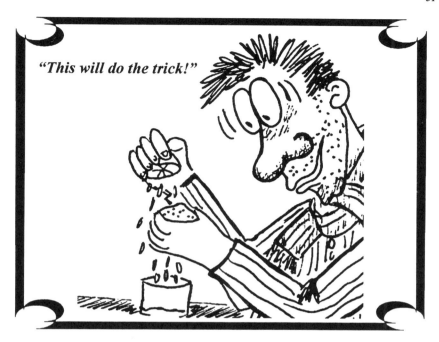

"*This will do the trick!*"

FEELING CHOKED - GOT A SORE THROAT?

Squeeze the juice from a lemon and sip slowly. Lemon is known to be an excellent medicinal fruit because of its multitude of healing properties. It is a good idea to consume it on a regular basis, especially in times of epidemics. Lemon is a great antiseptic. One obtains excellent results for mouth and throat inflammations.

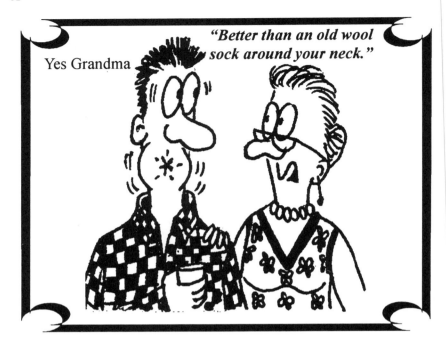

"Better than an old wool sock around your neck."

Yes Grandma

WHAT IS IT THIS TIME?

When it's not one thing, it's another! Inflammation of the tonsils (tonsillitis). Ah-ha, see what happens when you don't bundle up. Try this concoction: combine equal parts of water and garlic juice (About a tablespoon of each) and gargle several times during the day. (no need to swallow) Do me a favour will you? Don't complain about the taste of it..

Chapter IV

Physical Wear & Tear

Headaches
Insomnia
Muscle Aches (legs & knees)
Rheumatism

Sciatica
Stress (fatigue)
Weariness

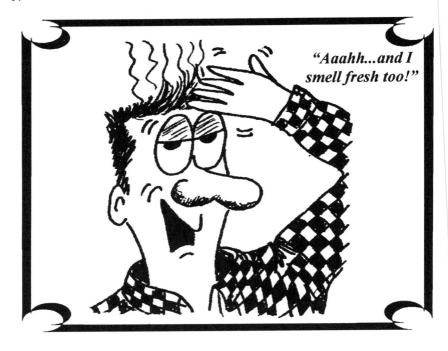

"Aaahh...and I smell fresh too!"

HERE'S A LITTLE HEADACHE FIGHTER

Did you know that rubbing a little bit of peppermint oil on your temples and forehead is known to alleviate some headaches. Avoid contact with your eyes when applying. A cooling sensation will be felt on applied areas and you'll find the odour of peppermint to be very soothing. Watery eyes and a runny nose may occur for a few minutes but will subside. Peppermint oil can be purchased in most natural and vitamin stores.

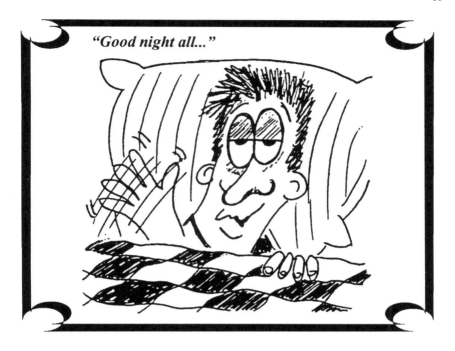

"Good night all..."

HONEY...I WANT MY MILK!

Had an active day and to make things worse you're having a difficult time falling asleep. Perhaps you ought to reconsider Grandma's advice.

At bedtime, drink the traditional glass of warm milk with a little honey.

Good night.

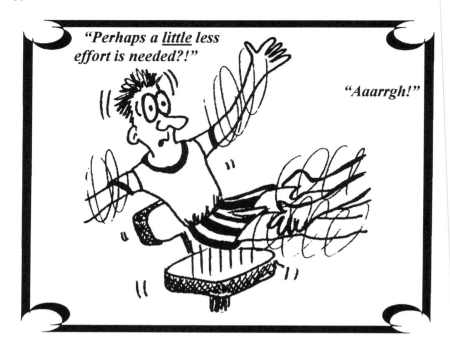

LOOKS LIKE YOU'RE SLOWING DOWN, CHAMP!

Yeah, I think the old legs and knees just don't have what it takes anymore. Well, well now, don't count them out yet. See if this helps you get back on track. A good, vigorous massage with camphor oil. Camphor is a medicine well-tried. Recommended for those aching, sore muscles. You must repeat this treatment as often as necessary, of course.

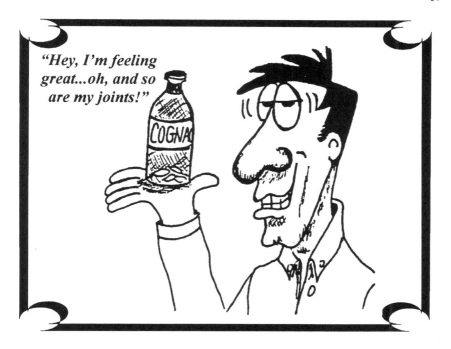

"Hey, I'm feeling great...oh, and so are my joints!"

LET'S KEEP THE DEVIL AWAY

Used since biblical times, garlic has been credited with many healing qualities and to this day, is still a universal remedy. Here is one sure way to alleviate rheumatism pain: skin the cloves of four large heads of garlic and marinate them in 450 ml of French brandy for ten days.

Now that it's ready, take half a teaspoon of the potion diluted in half a glass of water (room temperature) first thing every morning and notice the improvement within days.

When preparing this marinade, use a glass bottle and secure the top with foil paper to keep the strong odour in. Always keep the marinade at room temperature. Do not refrigerate. Do not eat the garlic cloves in the bottle.

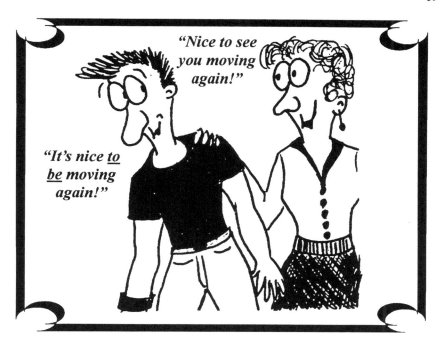

SOMEBODY HELP ME, PLEASE! NOT ANOTHER "SCIATICA" ATTACK...
(What a pain in the...back it can be)

In fact so much so, it even runs down the back of the thigh and leg causing direct pressure on a nerve. Now, now, no need to lose any sleep over it, as long as *you stretch and hold it!*

In order for the side to side stretch to be effective, you must first stand up straight with your feet slightly apart and holding a wrist or hand weight of two or three pounds. Lean towards the same side of the body as the weight. Retain this position for at least three minutes then do the other side.

Yes I know it's painful but it works by helping to unlock the compression on the nerve.

Left side, now try the right side! Aaahh...I feel better already.

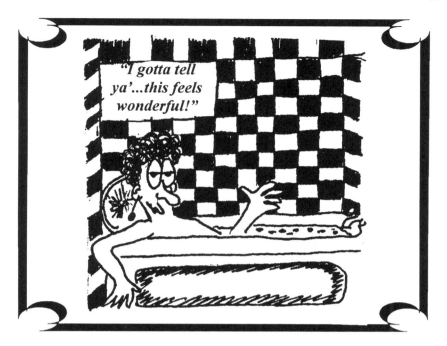

FATIGUE - STRESS
HECK, WE ALL SUFFER FROM IT AT ONE TIME OR ANOTHER

Give yourself a little time and find comfort in a cozy *"sage"* bath. Fill up the bathtub to which you'll add a good handful of *"sage leaves"*, wait a few minutes and soak right in there. Sage is known to have a decisive effect on making fatigue and stress symptoms disappear. *If sage leaves are not available, substitute a few drops of sage essential oil.*

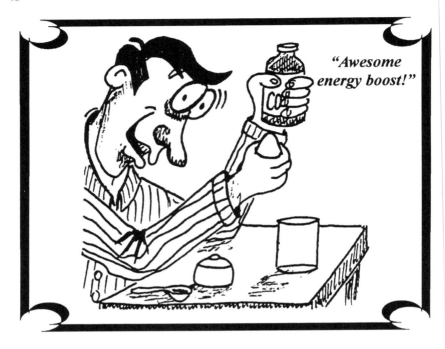

"Awesome energy boost!"

FEELING WEAK IN THE KNEES?

Try this energizing concoction. Use a blender. Mix two ounces of French cognac, one whole egg and two tablespoons of sugar. Blend until smooth and foamy. Cheers!

Chapter V

Bug Repellents

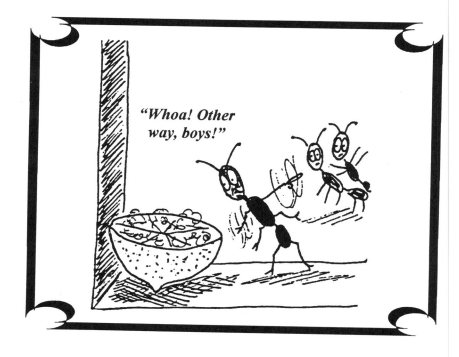

ATTACK OF THE ANTS...

Place half a moldy lemon in the invaded area and watch them march away.

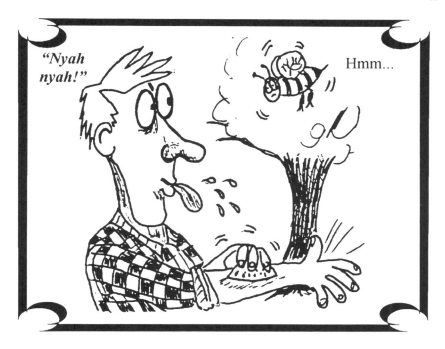

OUCH! GOT STUNG BY A BEE OR WAS IT A WASP?

If this is the case, first remove the stinger
then rub the area with lemon. Otherwise
use garlic or onion.
For mosquitos: rub parsley or leek.
For spiders: rub garlic or leek.

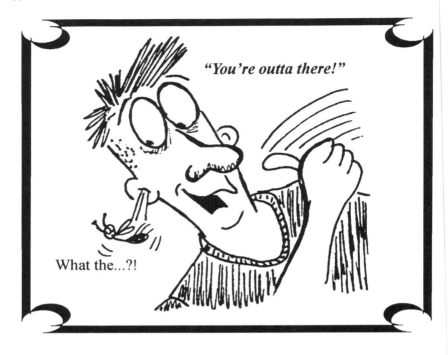

WHAT'S THE MATTER...GOT A BUG IN YOUR EAR?!

To expel the insect that found its way into your ear, insert a couple of drops of olive oil then tilt your head to the side and watch the insect slide out.

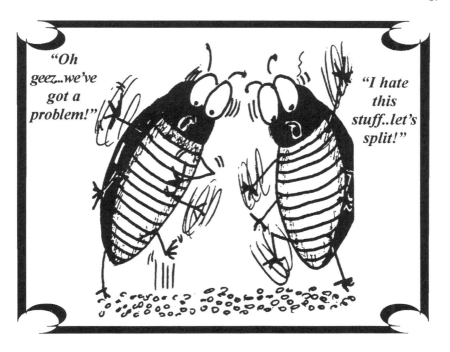

COCKROACHES - GODDAMN IT!

Whoever said you can't get rid of those nasty creepy crawlers? Here's for you buggers...by mixing the same amount of baking soda and sugar and then sprinkling generously all around the infested area, the chances are that the cockroaches will stop visiting your neighbourhood.
Got you!!

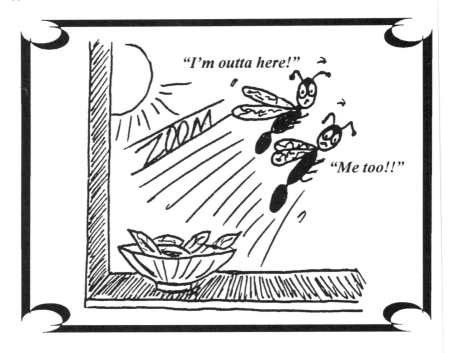

INVADED BY FLIES OR MOSQUITOS!?

On your window ledge place a small dish
of fresh basil. Stir up once in a while and
watch them fly away.
Fresh or dried eucalyptus leaves will also
do the trick.

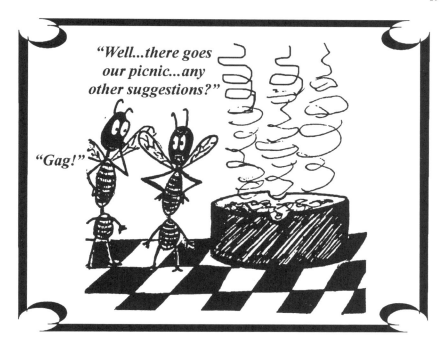

FINALLY...I CAN CAMP IN PEACE!

In an ashtray, burn some dried basil leaves. The smell of them will surely keep those sting-y insects out of your way.

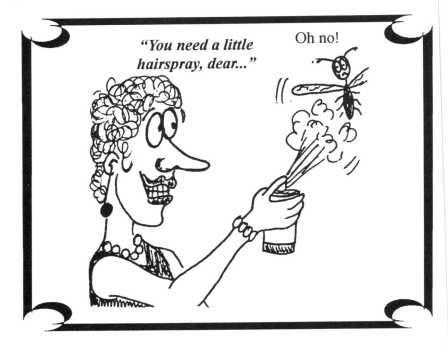

THOSE DARN BUGS REALLY BUG ME!

It's a bee...no it's a fly! Get me the hairspray and I'll stiffen the wings out of them!

This little trick is known to work quite effectively on most winged insects. If not, it will surely slow them down.

Chapter VI

Minor Illnesses

Cat Allergies

Colic (baby's colic)

Ear Ache

Hangover

Heartburn

Hiccups

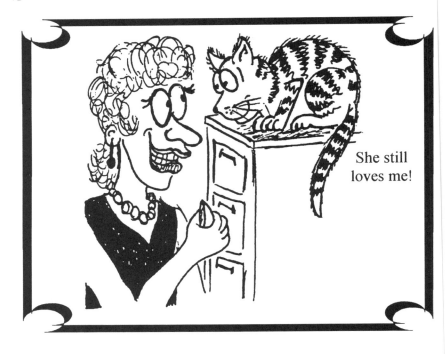

She still
loves me!

ALLERGIC TO YOUR FURRY FRIEND?

Eat half of a fresh mango every day and
sniffle no more.

If you plan on drinking the preserved
mango juice available at your local
grocery store, know that it won't be as
effective as the fresh fruit itself.

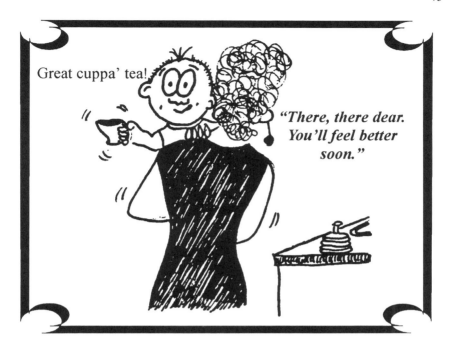

OH BABY-BABY, WHY ALL THE BIG TEARS FOR?

For your colicky* baby, prepare as you normally would for yourself a cup of fennel tea with a teaspoon of honey. Be sure to let the tea cool sufficiently before giving to the infant. The same tea is recommended and very soothing to babies on hot summer days.

* Colic is spasmodic abdominal pain.

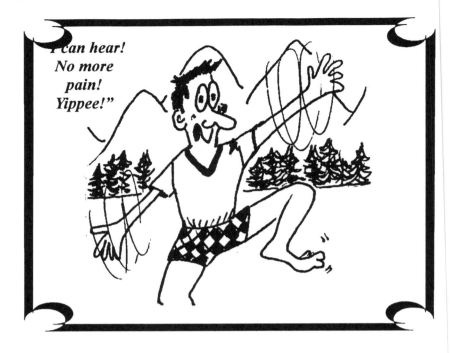

NOTHING LIKE A NASTY EAR ACHE, ESPECIALLY WHEN YOU'RE CAMPING IN THE MIDDLE OF NOWHERE

When needed, prepare a chamomile infusion, wait until lukewarm then mix with a little bit of olive oil. Insert a couple of drops into your ear, cover with a wad of cotton. Take a nap and wake up to the joys of the great outdoors.

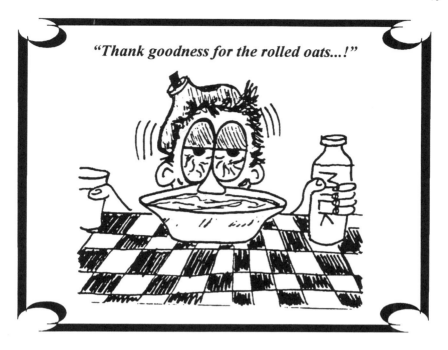

"Thank goodness for the rolled oats...!"

WHAT A PARTY! NOW PAY THE PRICE...
"HANGOVER"

Here is a suggested cure to consider.
On an empty stomach, eat a large bowl
of porridge mixed with milk and honey.
While the honey will give you a
temporary energy boost, the slow-
releasing carbohydrates in the oats re-
stabilizes your blood sugar level and the
milk will help neutralize acids.
Feel better?

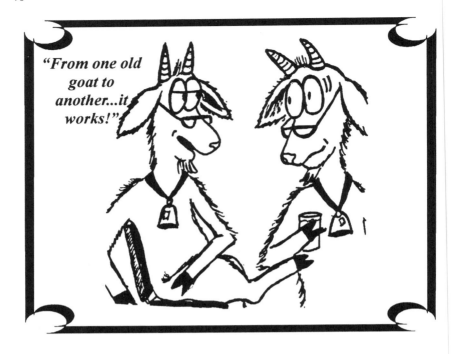

OH DEAR! I'D LOVE TO INDULGE BUT WHAT ABOUT MY HEARTBURN?

Well just for you, here's an old goat's advice!

Drink a half a cup or so of goat's milk two to three times a day. Whether you drink it before or after meals is really up to you. Whatever works best. Enjoy...

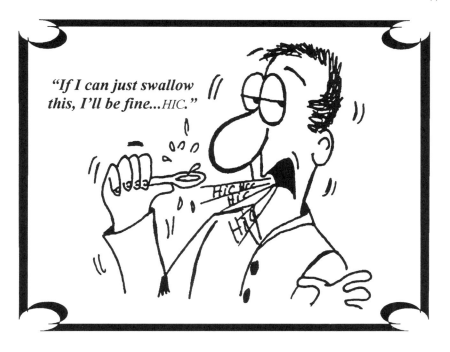

"*If I can just swallow this, I'll be fine...HIC.*"

HI! WHAT'S UP? "THE HICCUPS?"

Over indulgence can result in embarrassing bouts of hiccups but this formula has been reckoned to be a quick fix. Place a cube of sugar on a teaspoon and soak it in tarragon vinegar. Suck the sugar lump slowly and within a few minutes your hiccups will be gone. And it doesn't taste as bad as you might imagine.

Chapter VII

Tummy Ailments

Constipation

Diarrhea

Digestive (for stomach)

Intestinal Gas

Stomach Upset

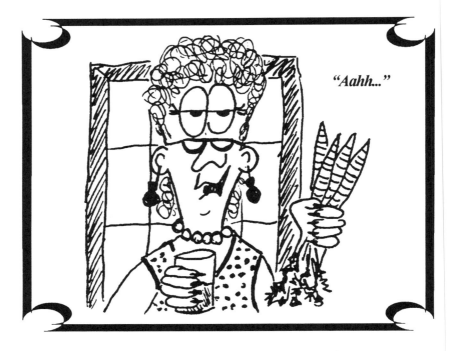

"Aahh..."

HAVING A HARD TIME?
DON'T PUSH YOUR LUCK!

Regular is the way to go so here are a couple of solutions.

Drink approximately half a glass of fresh carrot juice daily and you'll rid yourself of those nasty intestinal bugs.

Drinking half a glass of prune juice is also known to smooth the obstruction.

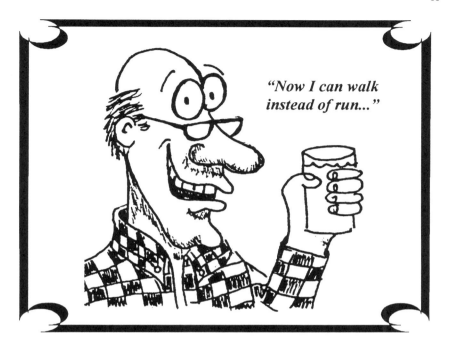

GOT THE RUNS?

For diarrhea consider a glass of bottled water (room temperature) with a tablespoon of sugar. Stir well and drink three to four times during the day.

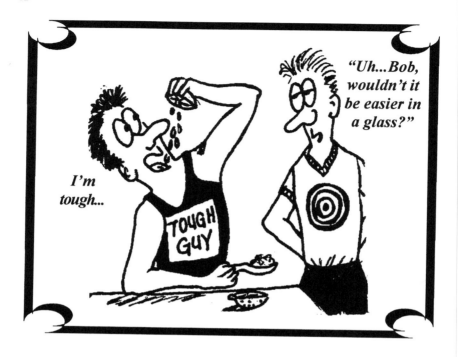

SOME PEOPLE JUST LIKE TO LEARN THINGS THE HARD WAY

Don't you know by now that there is a price to pay for abusing your stomach? Too much is just too much.

Well, try this if you don't want to stay with your head in the toilet all day. For a good stomach digestive, squeeze the juice of one lemon into a glass, add plenty of sugar and drink up.

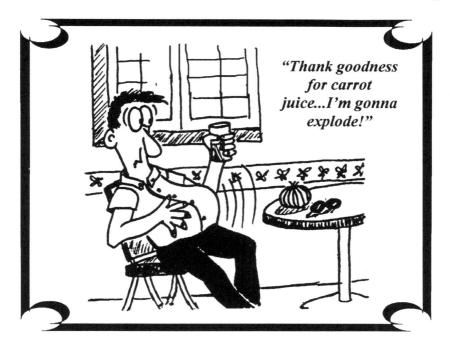

"Thank goodness for carrot juice...I'm gonna explode!"

LOOKS LIKE YOU SWALLOWED A LITTLE TOO MUCH AIR!

For a swollen abdomen due to intestinal gas accumulation, try eating raw onions or radishes. If that doesn't agree with your taste buds, a little fresh carrot juice after your meal will help release the contained gas.

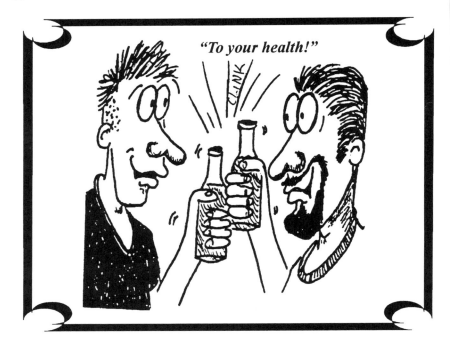

IS YOUR STOMACH FEELING UP TO NO GOOD? PERHAPS THAT FLU AGAIN!

Relieve your nasty discomfort with Coca-Cola Classic™ on ice. Sorry, but other soft drinks won't do the trick. Coke™ seems to act as a stomach cleanser and the sparkling fizz that makes you burp will also make you feel better.
Coke is it!™

Chapter VIII

Summer Hazards

Hay Fever
Heat Exhaustion
Thirst Suppressor

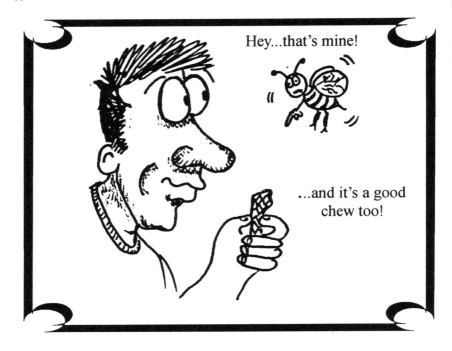

SPRING HAS SPRUNG AND SO HAVE THE ALLERGIES

Whether the causes are environmental, pollens, foods, dusts or microorganisms consider chewing on half a teaspoon of honeycomb after breakfast or before heading out the door.

Chew the honeycomb as though it was a piece of gum. After five or ten minutes of doing so, spit out the wax.

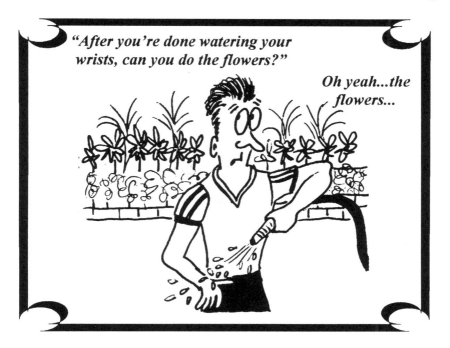

COOL DOWN, CHUM! A LITTLE COMMON SENSE IS ALL IT TAKES

If the summer heat is melting you down, cooling off is as easy as turning on the tap and letting the cold water run on your wrists. You'll feel refreshed within moments. Do repeat this action as often as needed.

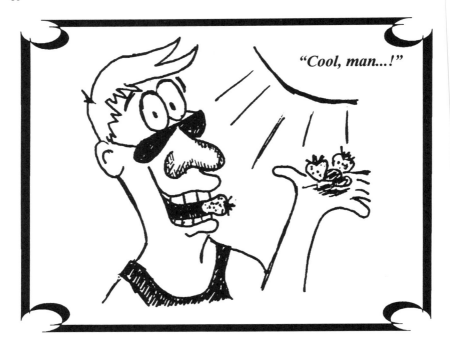

CAN'T STAND THE HEAT?!?

To quench your thirst during those hot summer days, eat wild strawberries or red currants (gooseberries).

Chapter

IX

Unwanted Body Odours

Bad Breath
Foul Shoe Odours
Sweaty & Smelly Feet

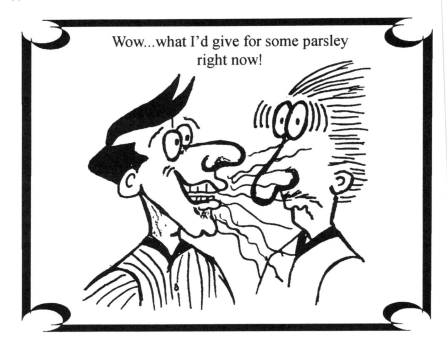

TALK TO YOU LATER

In case of bad breath, chew on a little fresh parsley or drink peppermint tea after your meal.

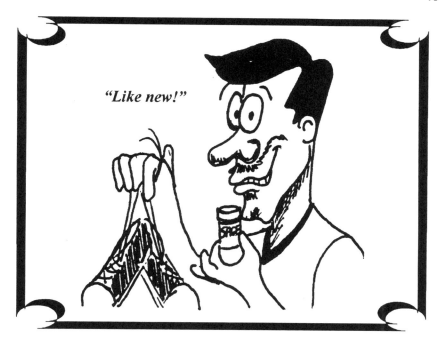

HEY BUDDY, A NEW PAIR OF SHOES WOULDN'T HURT!

True enough, but you're afflicted with the tight wallet syndrome. To take care of this offensive odour, sprinkle the inside of your shoes with a little sage powder.

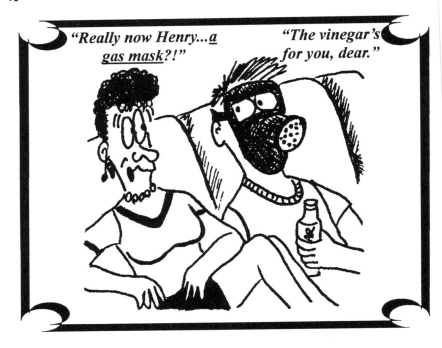

IF YOU THOUGHT SWEATY FEET WERE BAD...WHAT ABOUT SWEATY <u>AND</u> SMELLY?

Either of the above is enough to spoil what could have been a perfect date. Worry no more, my friend! Sit back and relax. Simply bathe your feet in a basin of warm water to which you've added a half cup (or so) of white vinegar. Repeat as frequently as necessary. For some perhaps daily, while for others two or three times a week may suffice. You be the judge.

Chapter X

Travelling Disorders

Airplane Ear
Motion Sickness

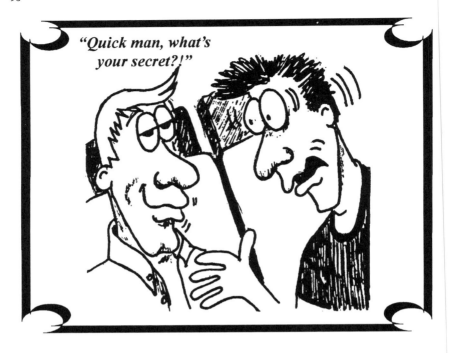

FEELING THE PRESSURE?

"Airplane Ear" as it is called, caused by airplane cabin pressure, can be prevented by simply chewing gum. It keeps you swallowing and keeps your eustachian (auditory) tubes open.

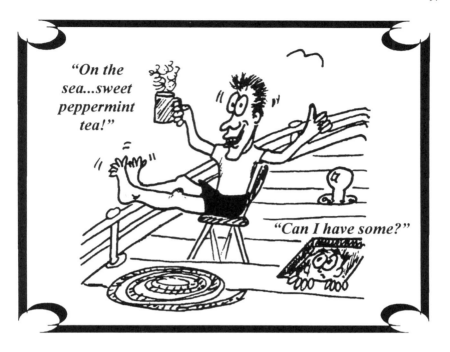

ALL THIS TRAVELLING IS MAKING ME FEEL RATHER QUEASY!

In case of motion sickness, peppermint tea will soothe and calm your stomach. Nibbling on whole grain crackers is equally helpful. Make sure you stay cool. When travelling by car, roll down a window. If you're sailing, stand on deck. Now, if you're flying, open the overhead vent.

Quick Fix Chest of Home-made Remedies

Play it safe and try to have the following ingredients on hand:

Apple Cider Vinegar

Baking Soda
Basil (dried)
Bubble Bath Soap

Camphor Oil
Castor Oil
Chamomile Tea
Chewing Gum
Coca-Cola™
Cotton Gloves
Cayenne Pepper

Eucalyptus Oil

French Cognac
Fennel Tea

Hair Spray
Honeycomb

Laurel Leaves
Liquid Honey
Linseed Oil

Marshmallows

Olive Oil

Peppermint Oil
Peppermint Tea
Prune Juice

Red Wine
Rolled Oats
Rubbing Alcohol

Sage Powder (leaves & essential oil)
Salt
Sugar (cubes and granular)
Sweet Almond Oil

Tarragon Vinegar

Vitamin E Soap
Vitamin E Oil

Water (bottled)
Witch Hazel Solution
White Vinegar
Whole Grain Crackers

List continued next page

Fresh ingredients as required:

Apples

Basil (fresh)

Carrot Juice
Cherries (fresh or dried)
Cucumber

Eggs

Figs

Garlic
Goat's Milk

Leeks
Lemons

Milk
Mango

Onions

Parsley (fresh)
Plain Yogurt
Potatoes

Radishes
Red Currants (gooseberries)

Strawberries

About the Author...

Viviane Kolp was born in Arlon, Belgium, a little town only steps away from Luxembourg. She is the fourth of eight children, four brothers and three sisters.

Her family emigrated to Canada in 1969 and lived in Montreal until their move to Vancouver in 1978. Her father passed away in 1986.

Viviane's languages include: French, English, Luxembourg (dialect) and German. She attended classical ballet school from early childhood to young adulthood.

Ms. Kolp holds a diploma in Modern Massage, certificates in Practical Massage, Human Anatomy & Physiology, Medical Terminology, Psychology & Social Work and is a Certified Pharmaceutical Assistant.

She has been an independent massage therapist for the past twenty years, the last fifteen have been in private practice.

Viviane lives with her mother who is her greatest supporter. They have a very special and close relationship. Together, as always, they have teamed up once again to share their delightful collection of sweet and sour pain-free remedies that were used in days past and have endured the test of time.

Acknowledgements...

I wish to express my deep and lasting appreciation to my mother, Yvette Scheuer, for her constant encouragement and for all her subsequent guidance. To Diana V. Van Baaren for her inspired cartoons. To my mother's sister Rosy for contributing many old remedies.

Finally, my sincere gratitude to my mother's brother, Joseph (Josy), for his reliable help and inspiration.

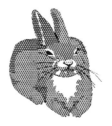

Nature's Delight

Of its roots
dreams the tree
that sleeps.
Ignored
are the silent screams
of those
whose pain is deep.
Pure
are the streams
that flow
embedded in nature's glow.
Energized
by sunlit beams
that give us light
warmth at night
and power to grow.